# Cancer Can't Stop Me: A Stress Relieving Cancer Coloring Book

Hi everyone,

Thank you so much for purchasing this coloring book. I hope you enjoy it!

I have a special surprise for you...

**Claim your gift here: https://bit.ly/2K58AtH**

Thanks so much and happy coloring!

# Color Test Page

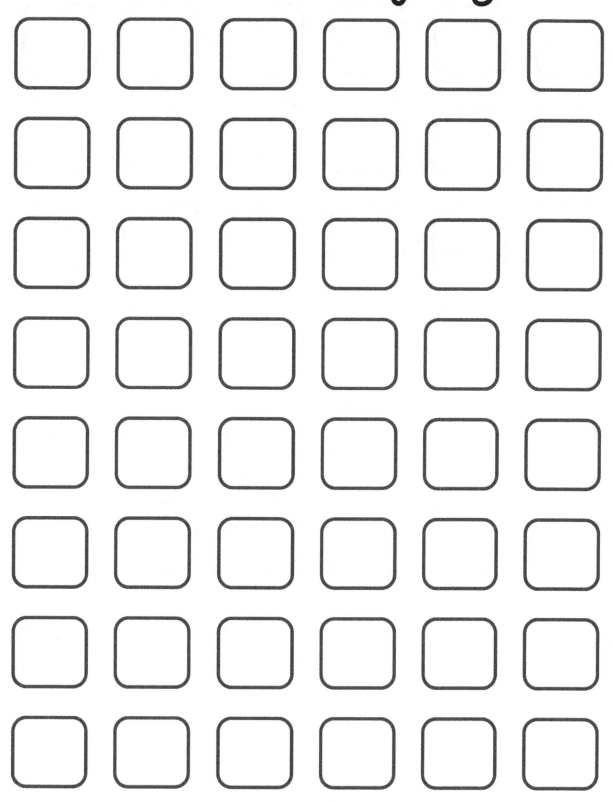

# Color Test Page

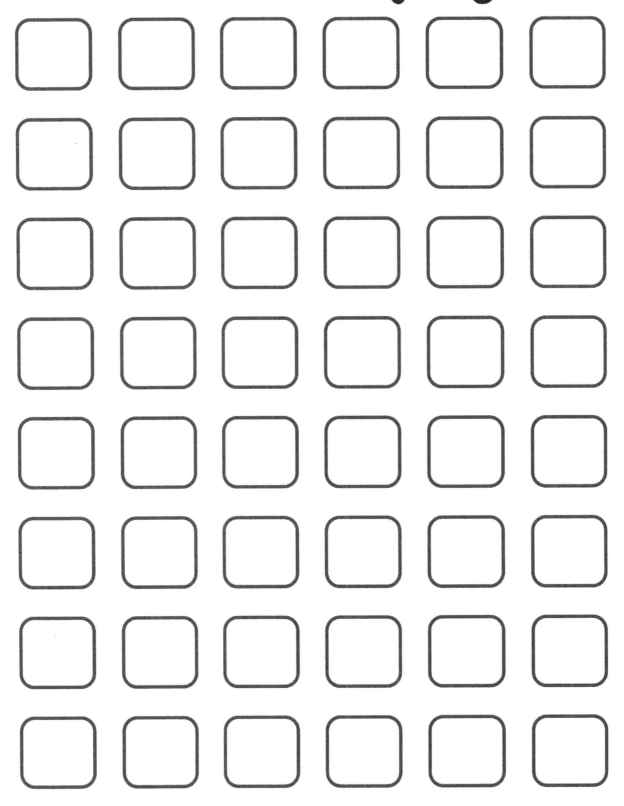

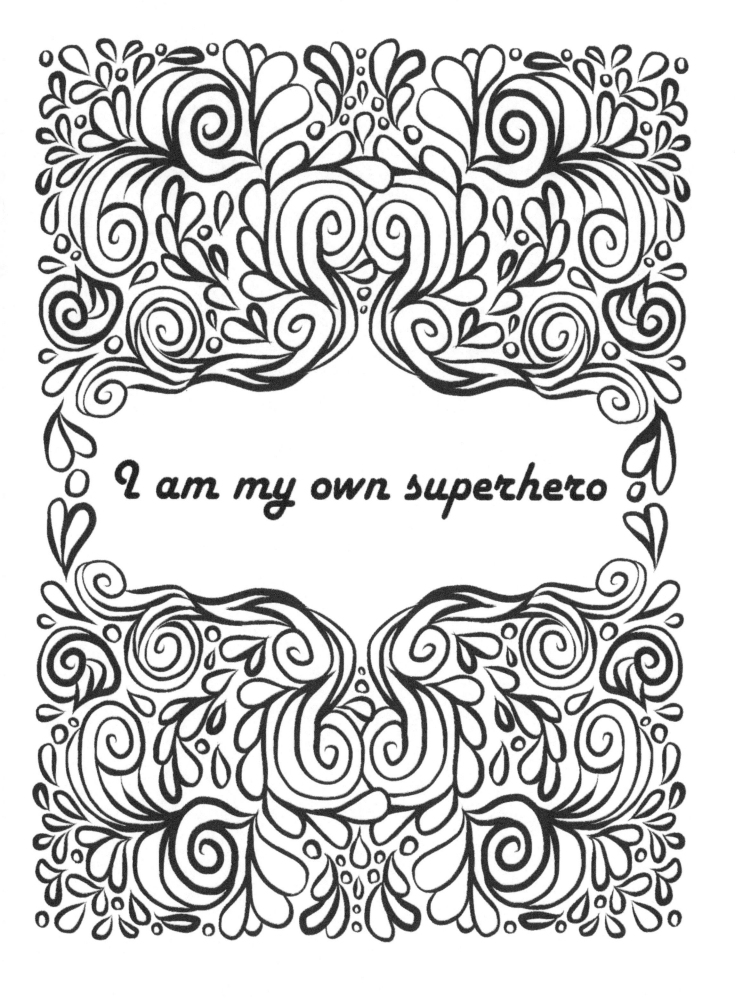

I am my own superhero

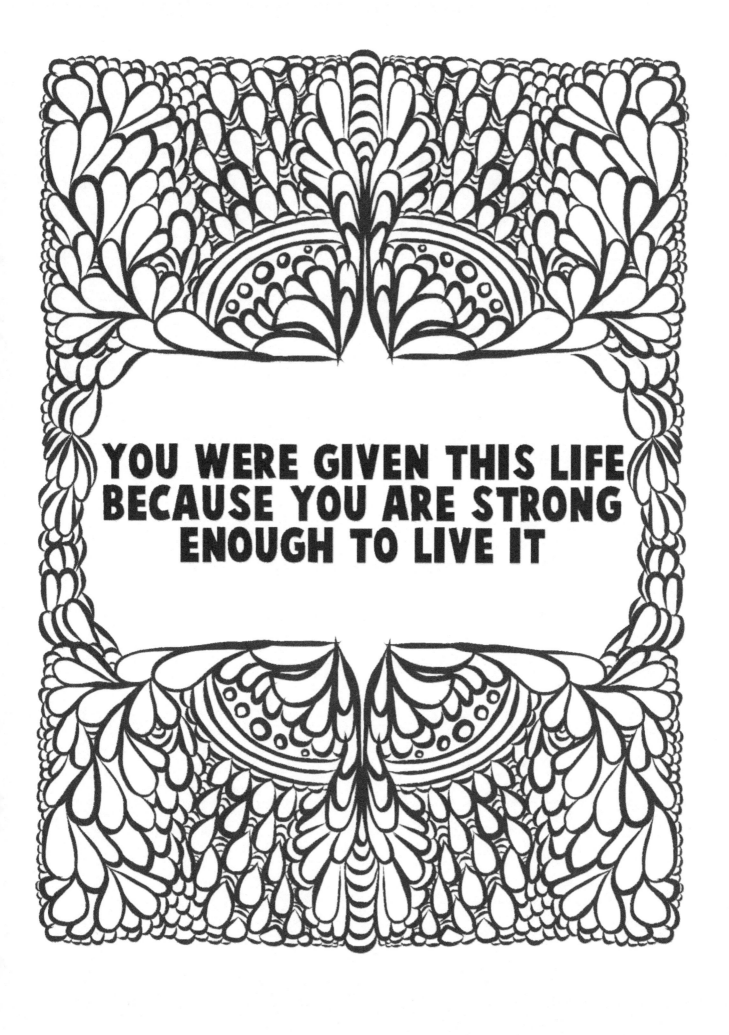

YOU WERE GIVEN THIS LIFE BECAUSE YOU ARE STRONG ENOUGH TO LIVE IT

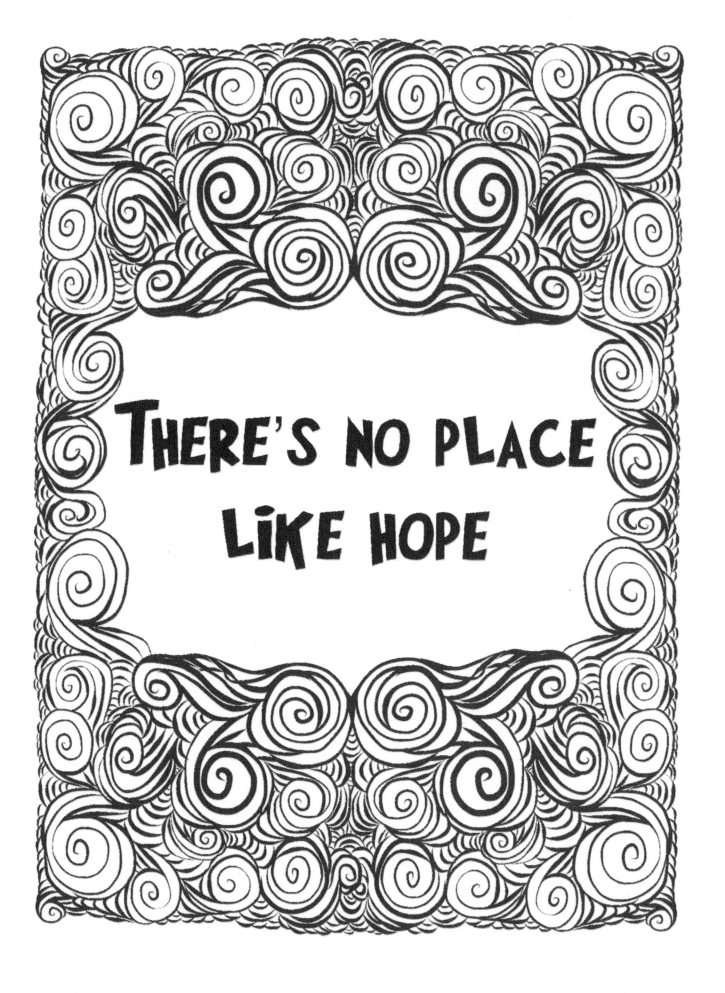

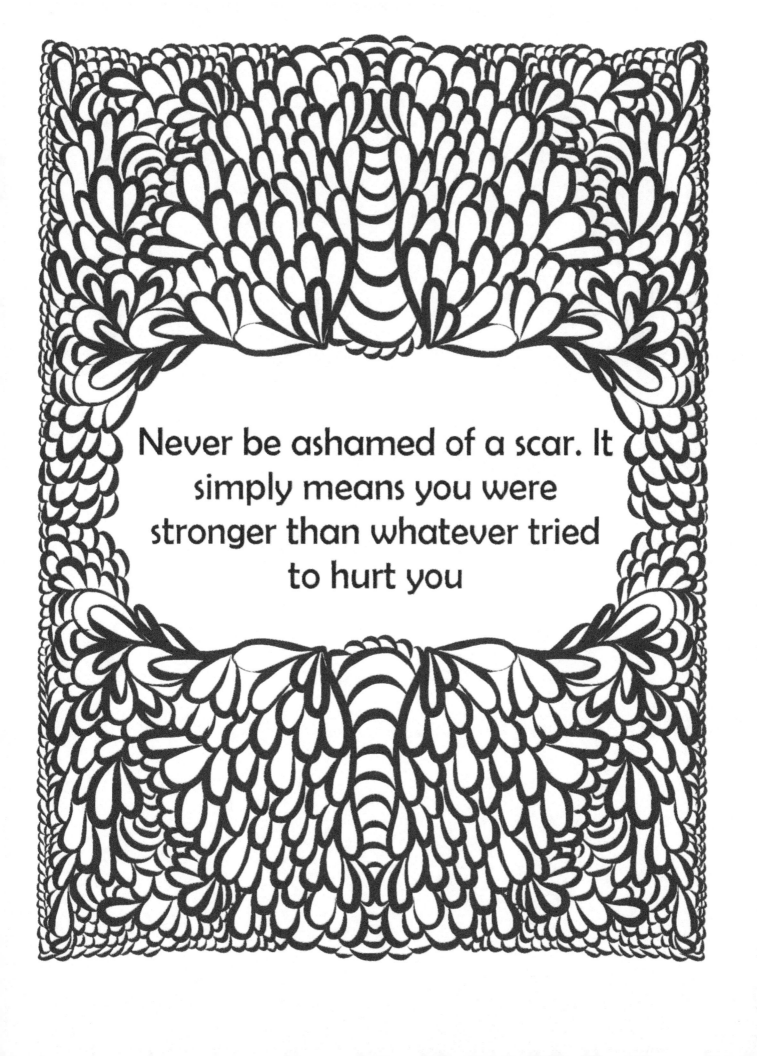

Never be ashamed of a scar. It simply means you were stronger than whatever tried to hurt you

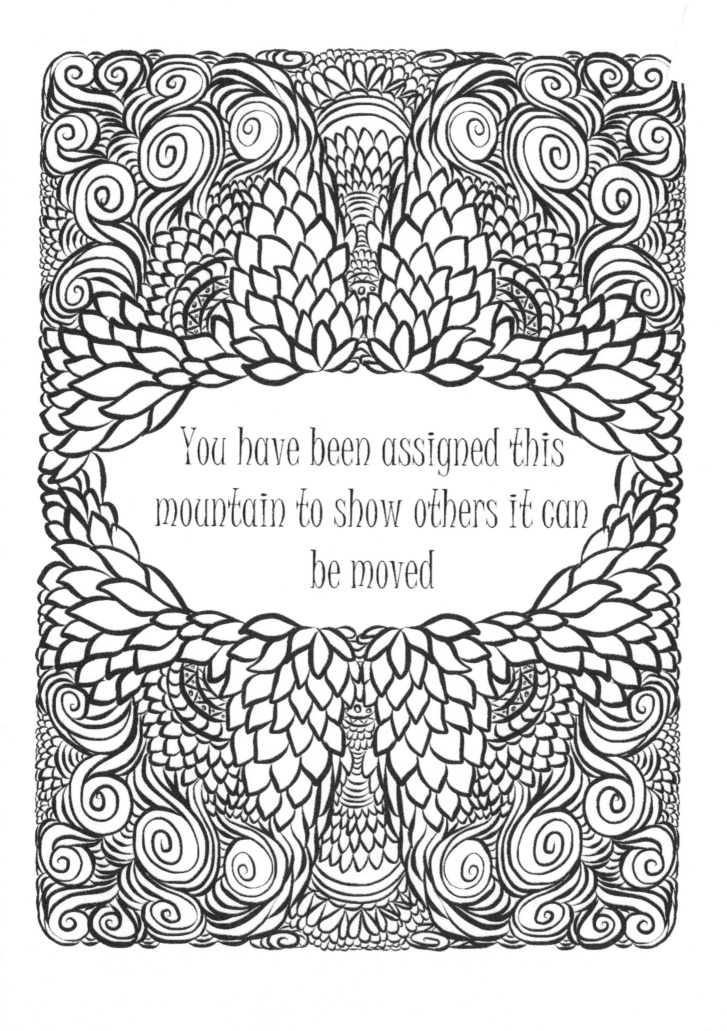

You have been assigned this mountain to show others it can be moved

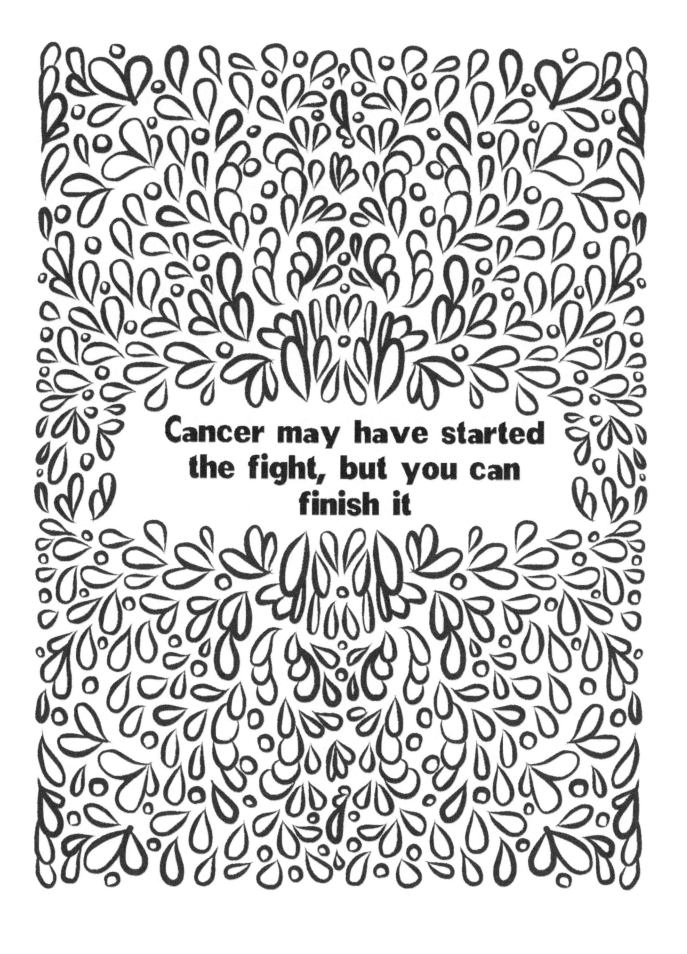

Cancer may have started the fight, but you can finish it

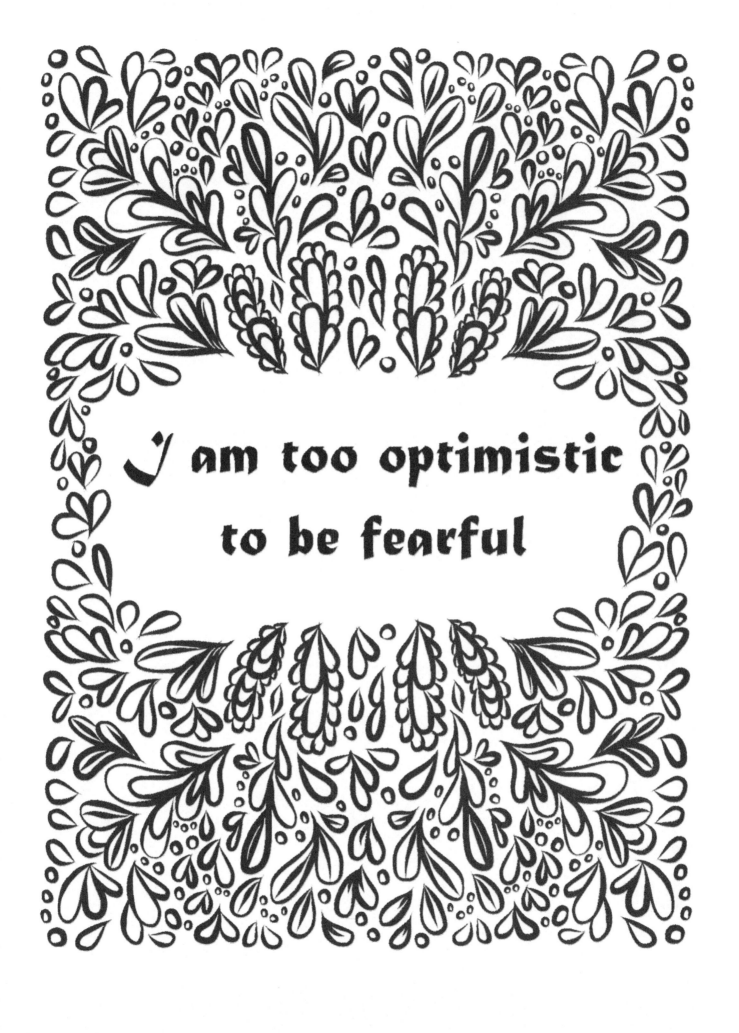

I am too optimistic
to be fearful

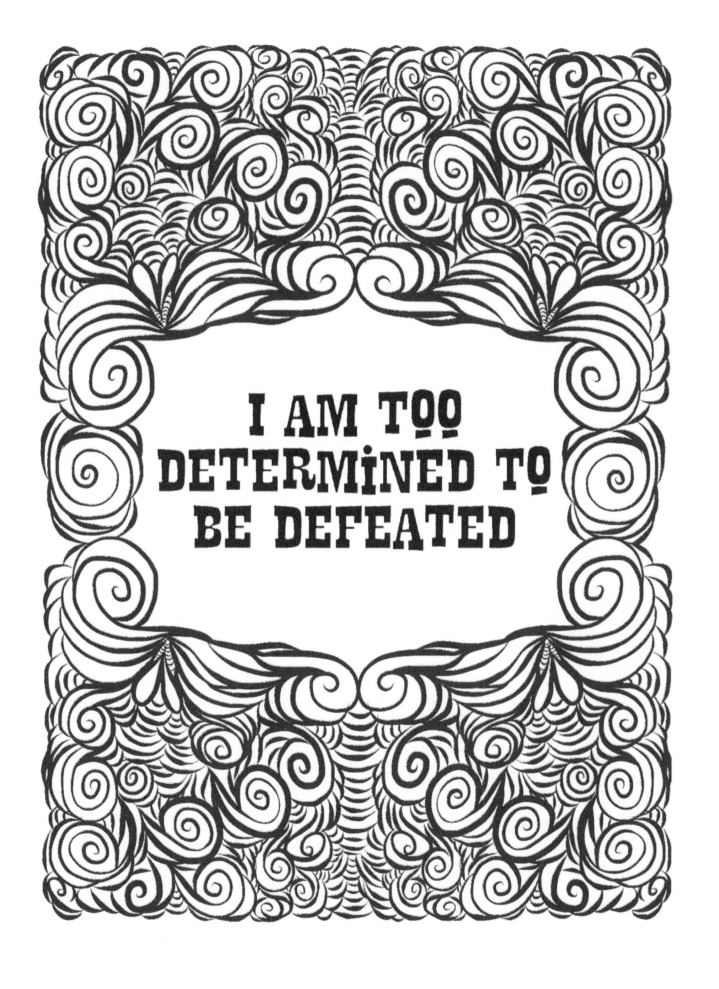

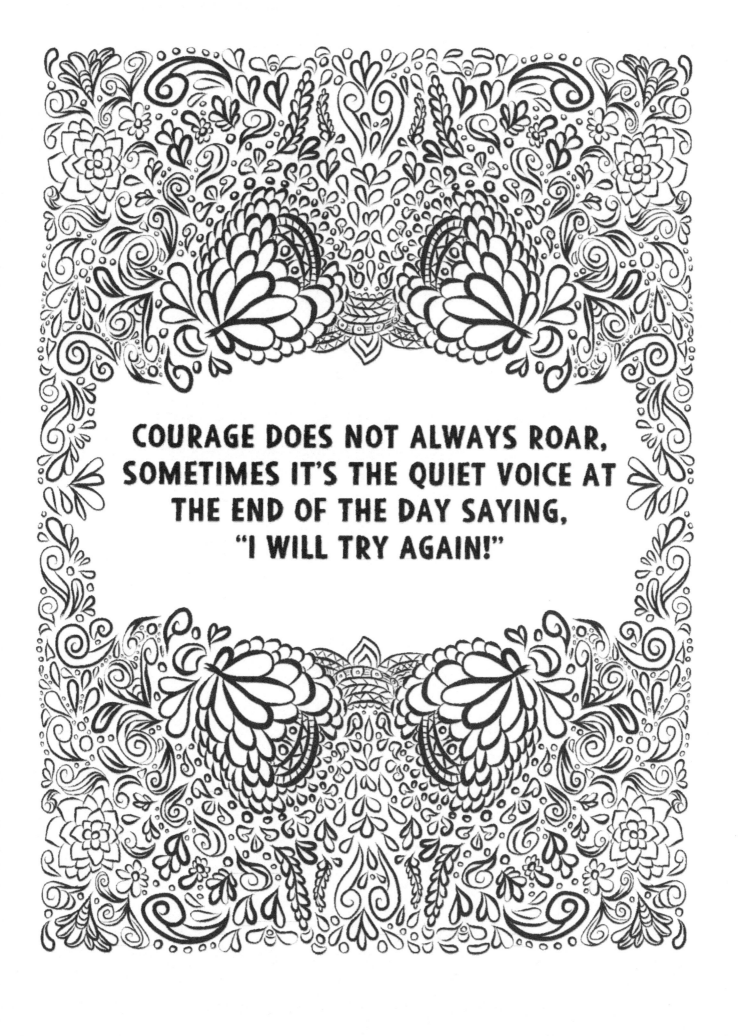

COURAGE DOES NOT ALWAYS ROAR,
SOMETIMES IT'S THE QUIET VOICE AT
THE END OF THE DAY SAYING,
"I WILL TRY AGAIN!"

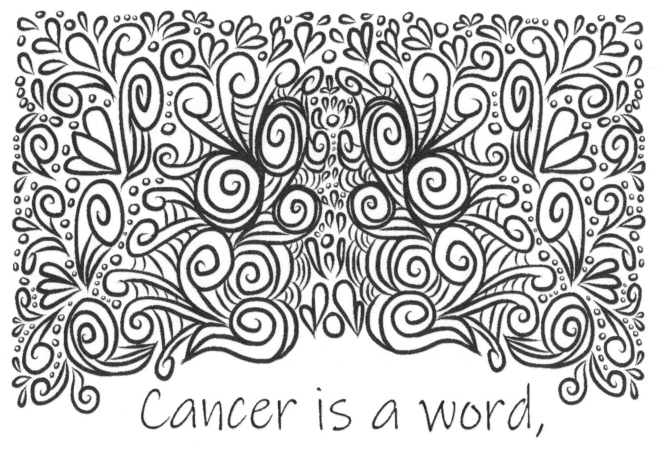

Cancer is a word,
not a sentence

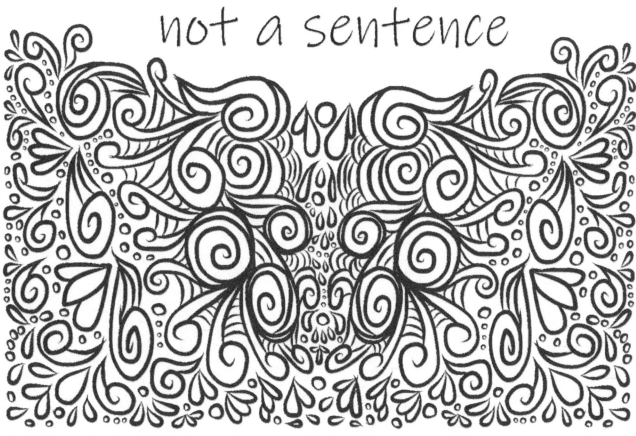

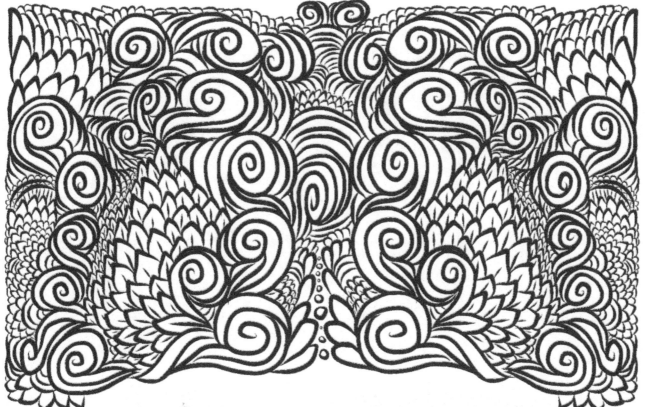

# I AM STRONG

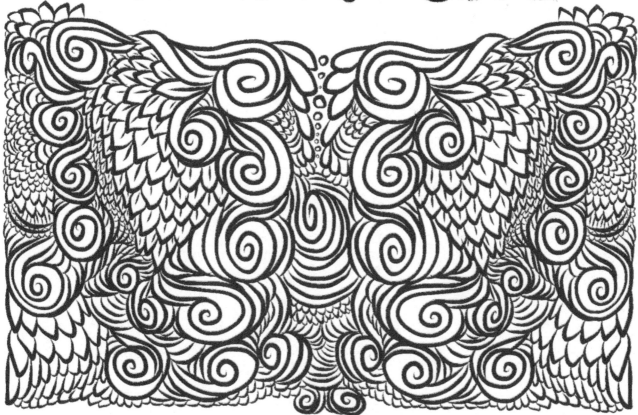

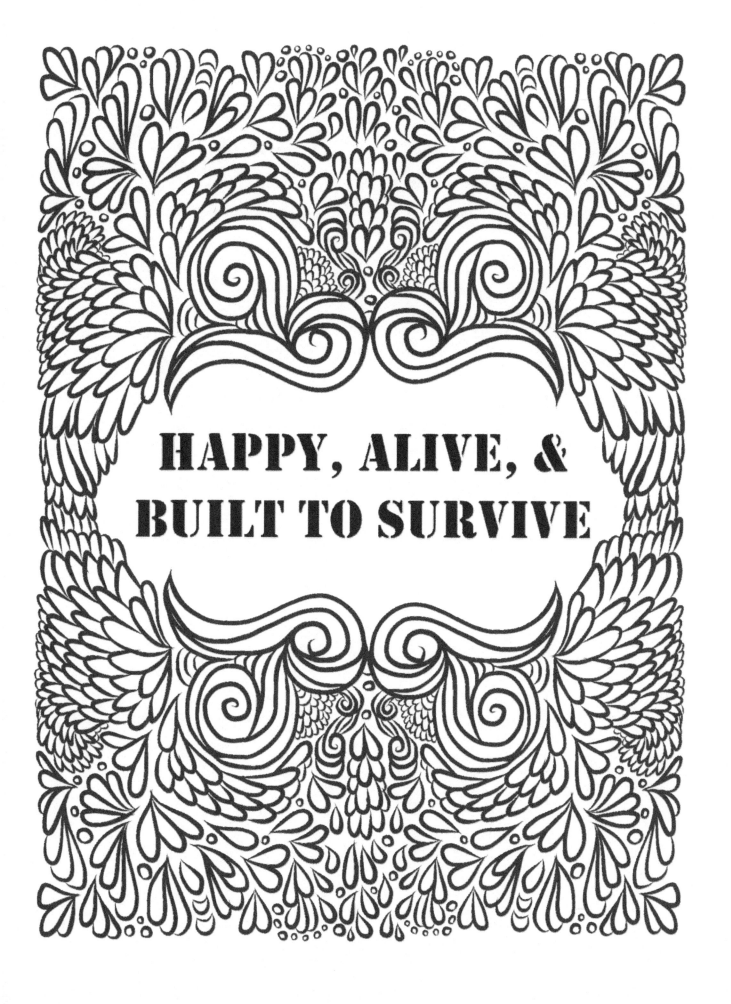

HAPPY, ALIVE, &
BUILT TO SURVIVE

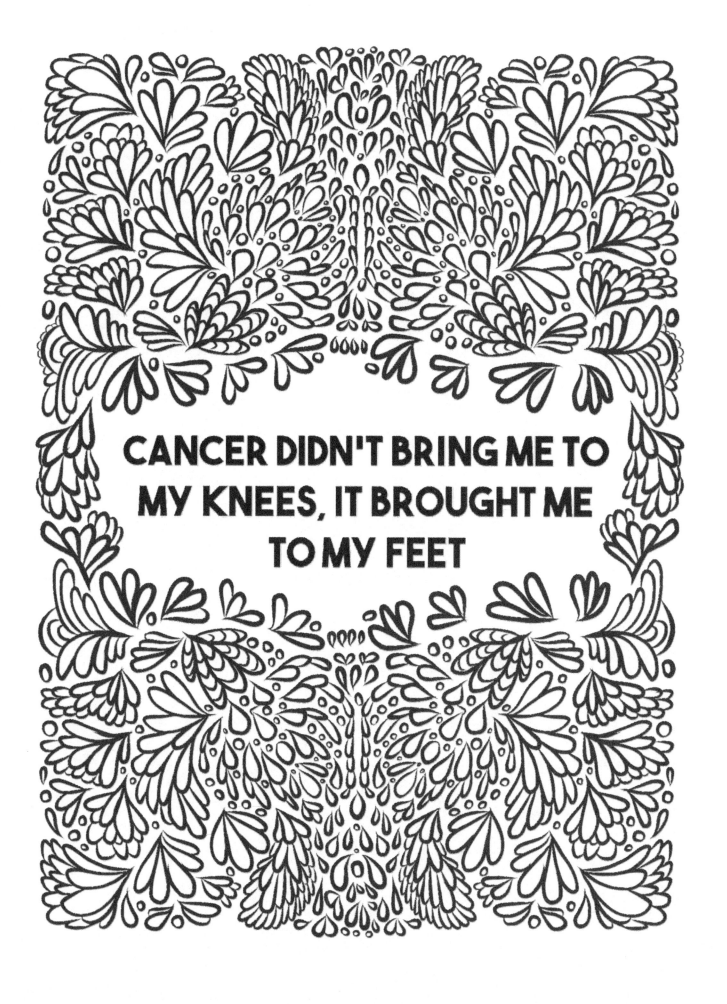

CANCER DIDN'T BRING ME TO
MY KNEES, IT BROUGHT ME
TO MY FEET

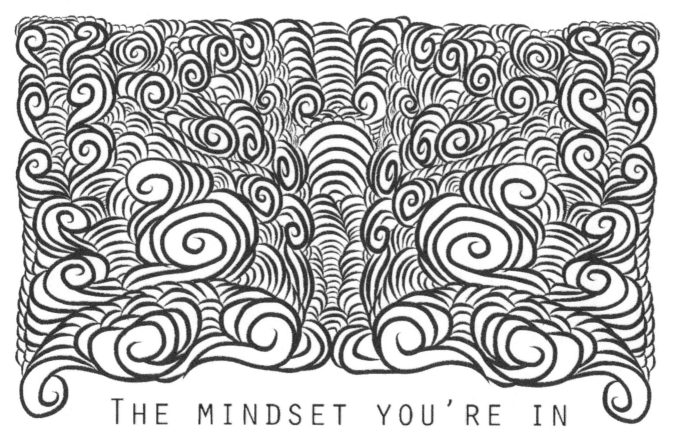

THE MINDSET YOU'RE IN
IS THE BIGGEST WEAPON
YOU HAVE

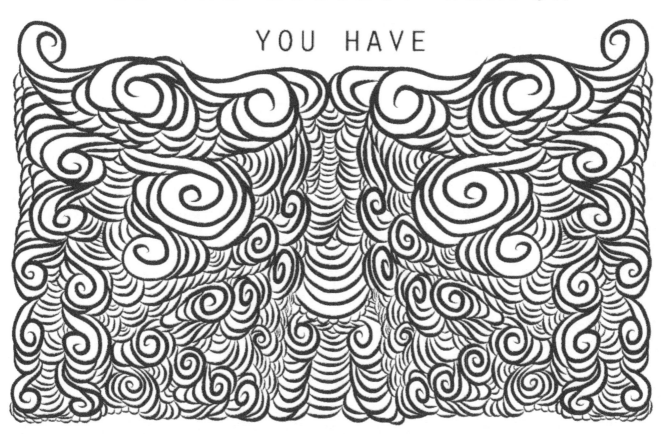

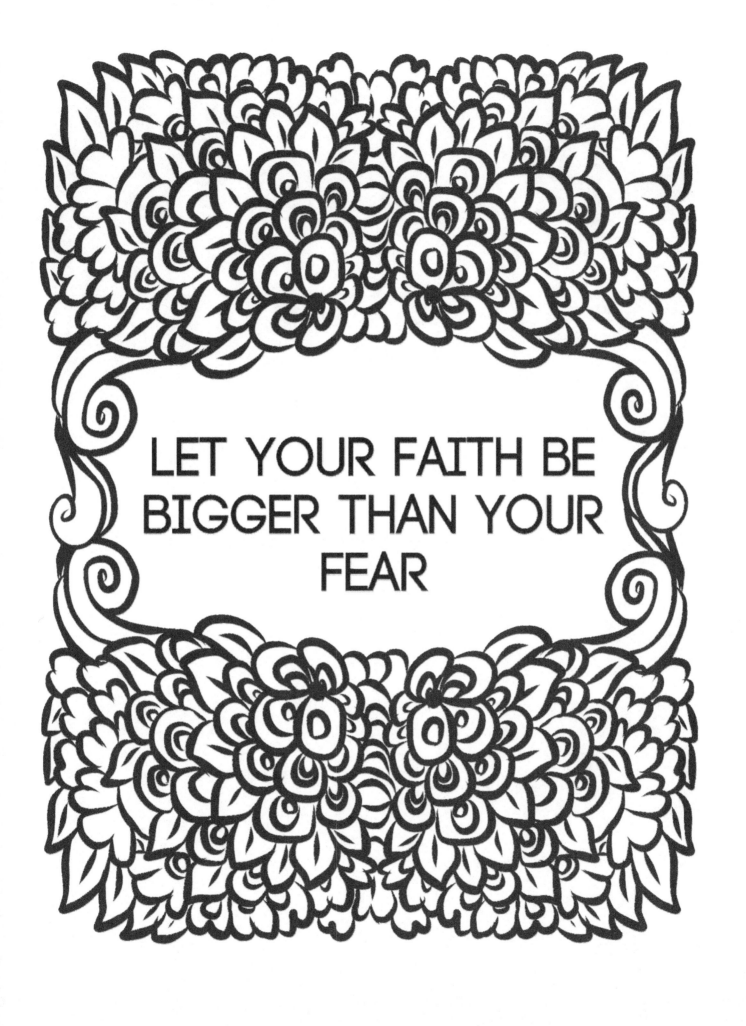

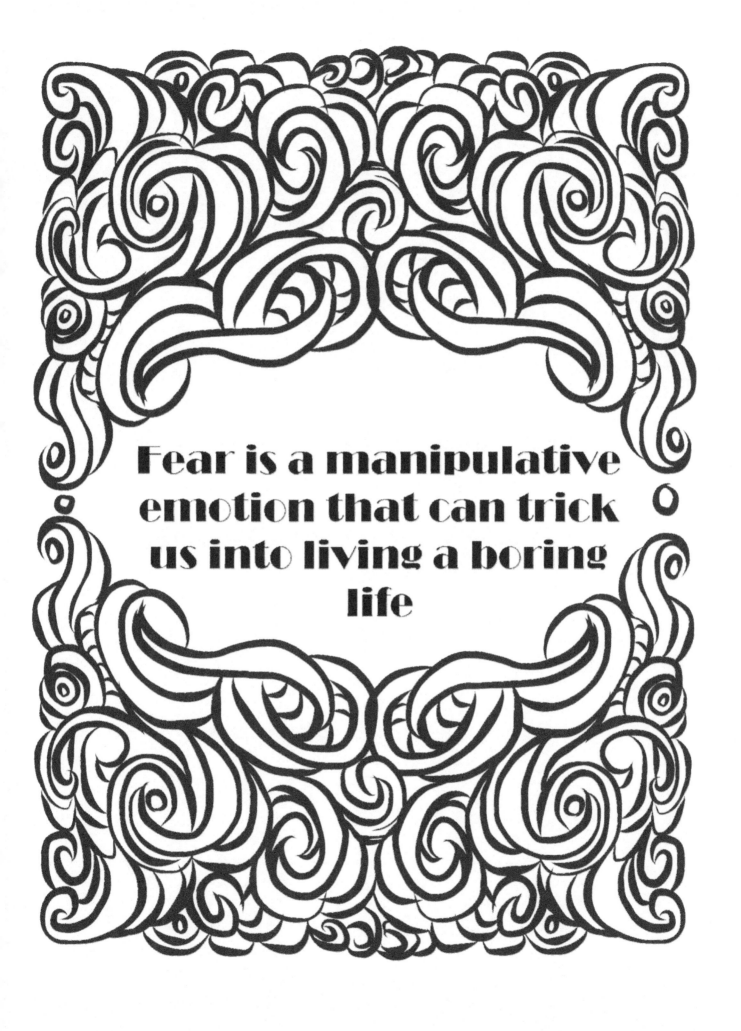

Fear is a manipulative emotion that can trick us into living a boring life

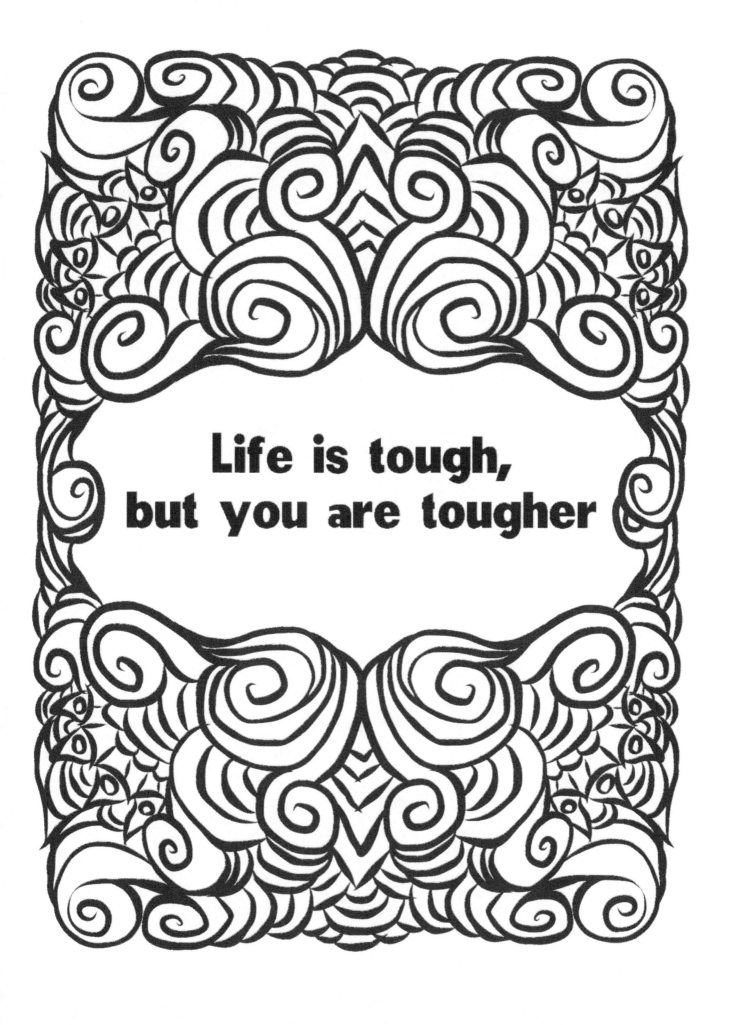

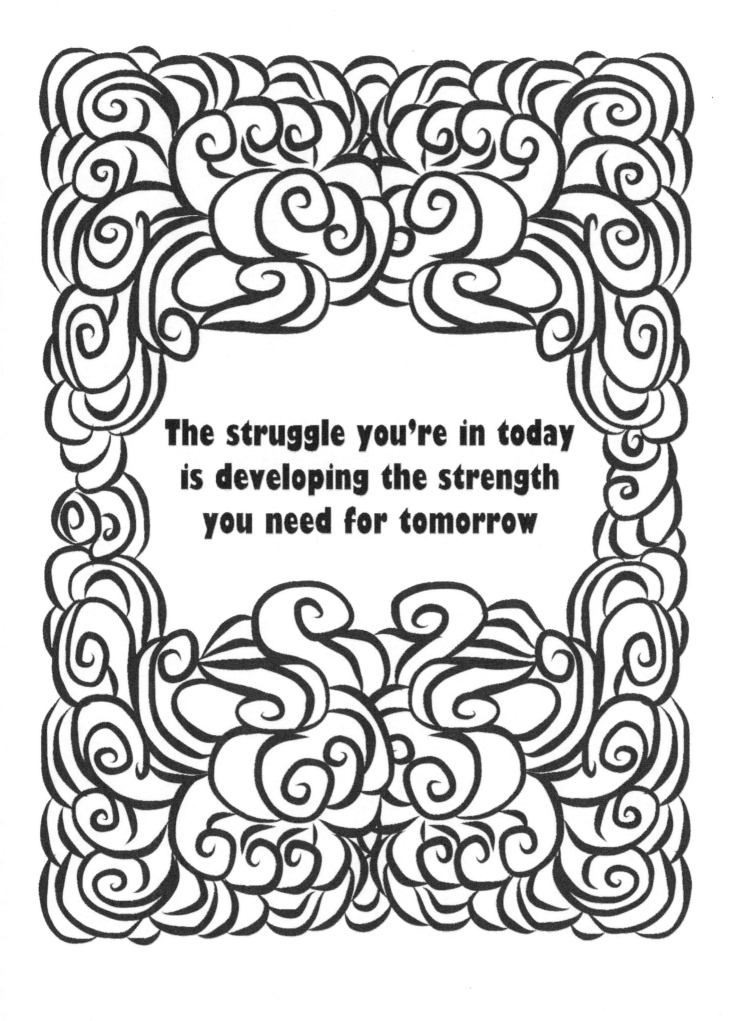

The struggle you're in today
is developing the strength
you need for tomorrow

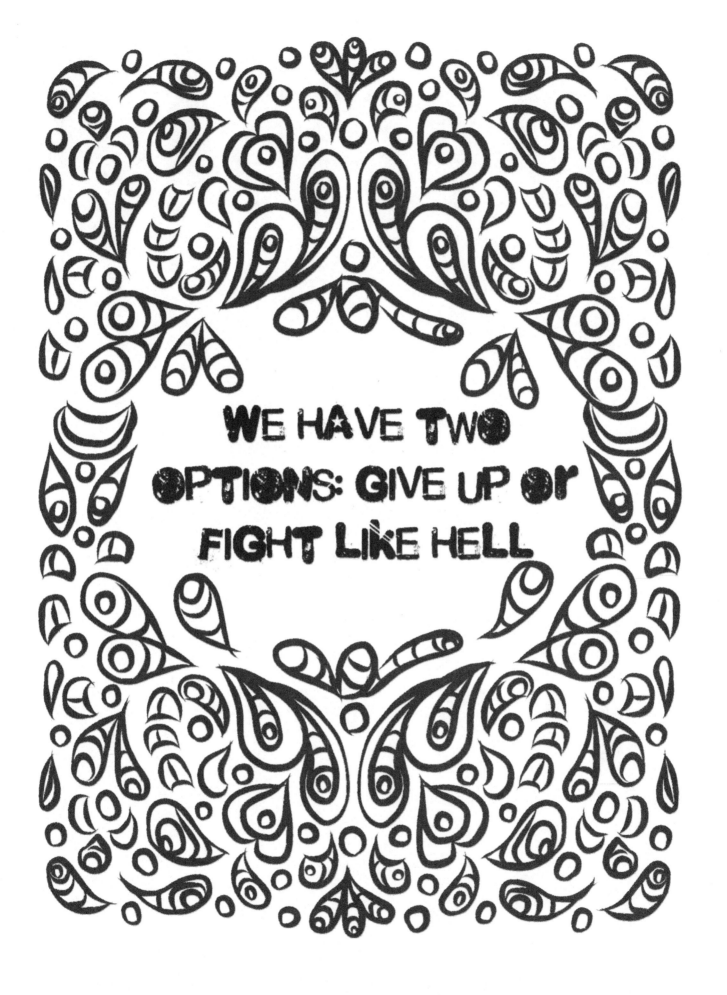

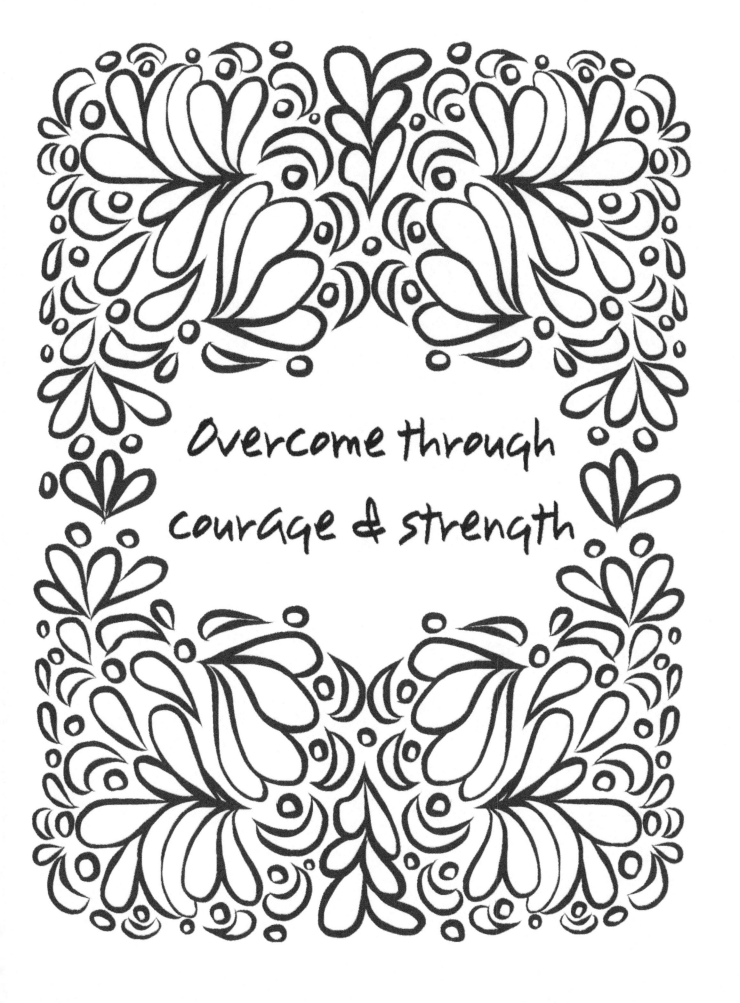

Overcome through courage & strength

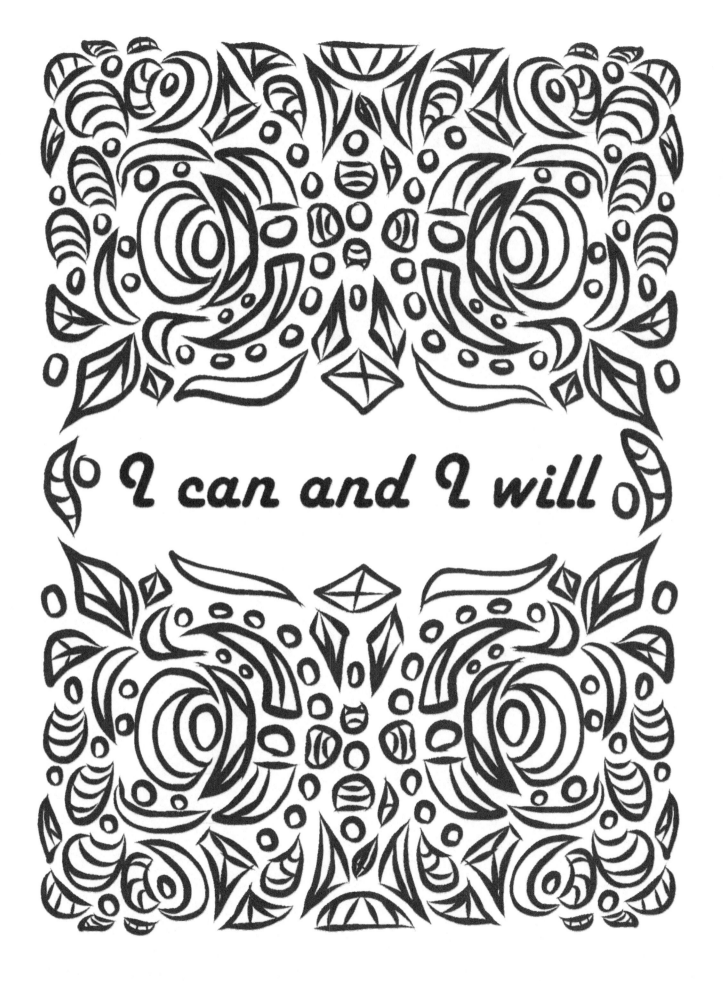

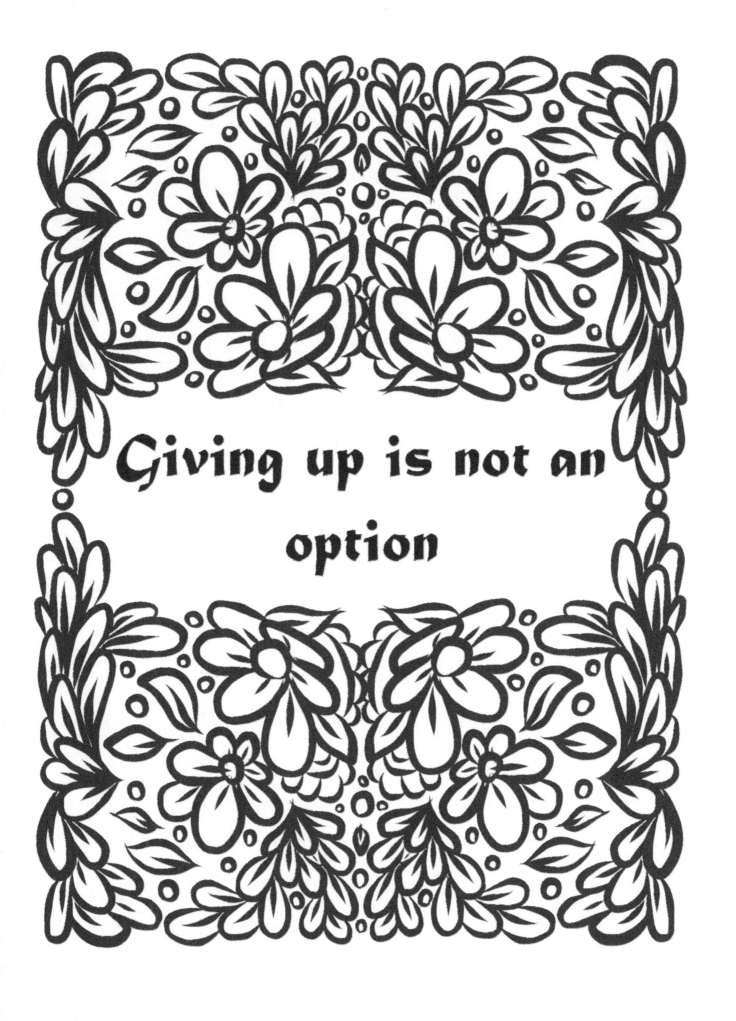

Giving up is not an option

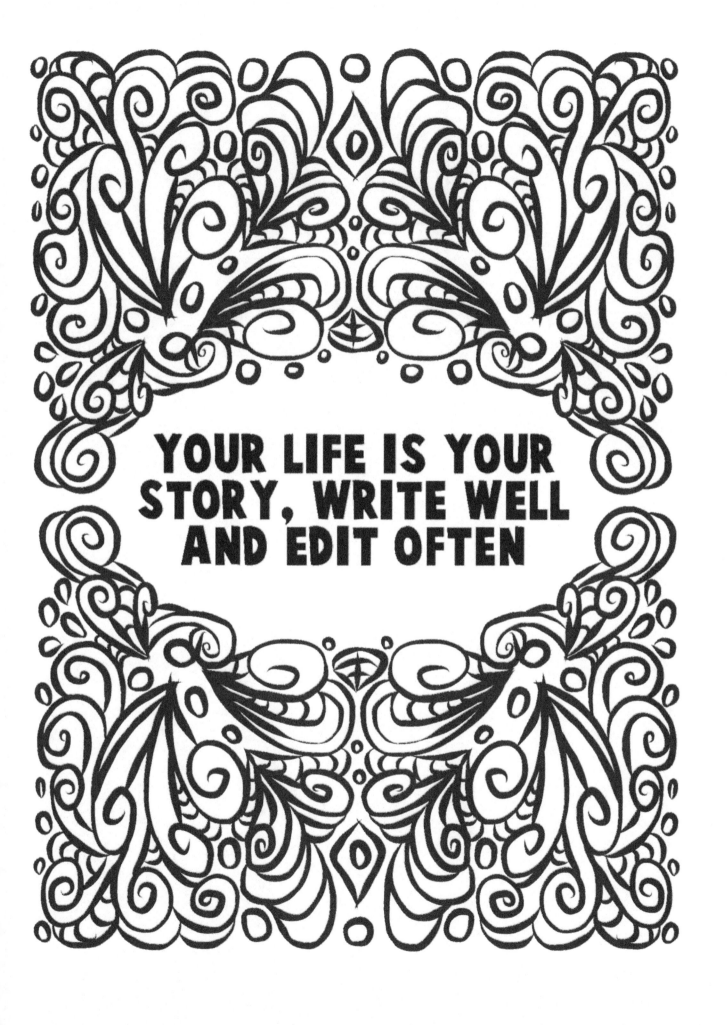

YOUR LIFE IS YOUR STORY, WRITE WELL AND EDIT OFTEN

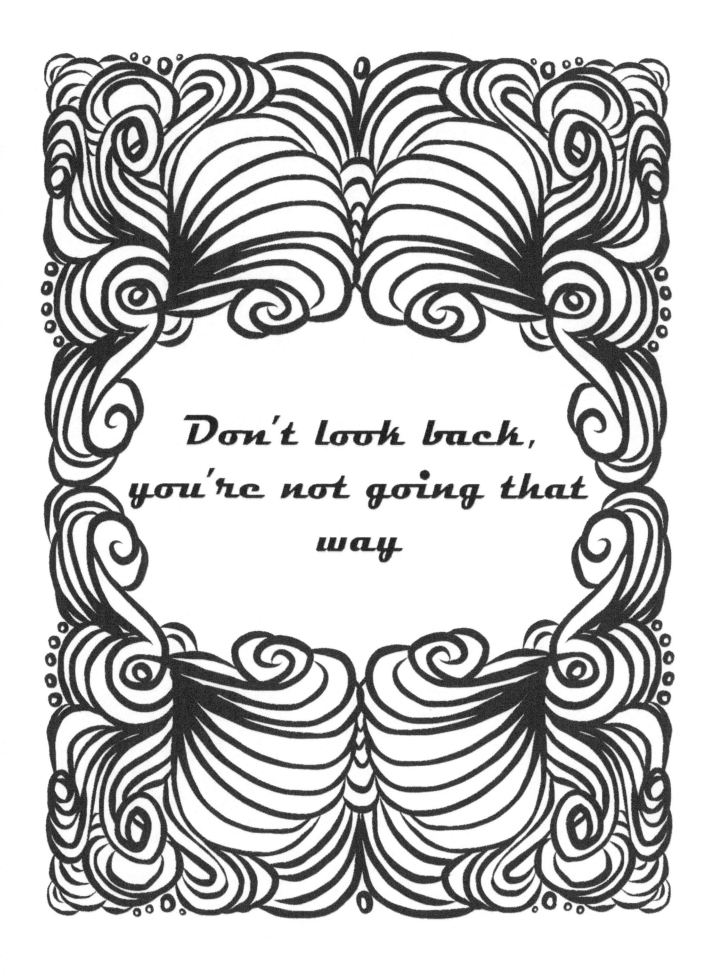

Don't look back, you're not going that way

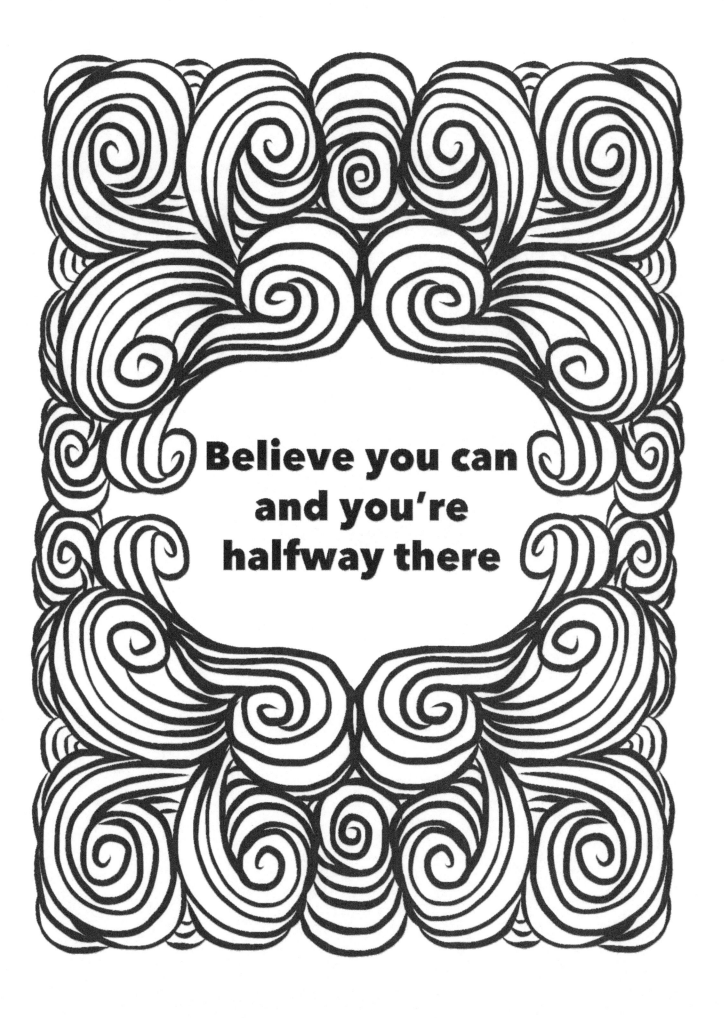

Believe you can and you're halfway there

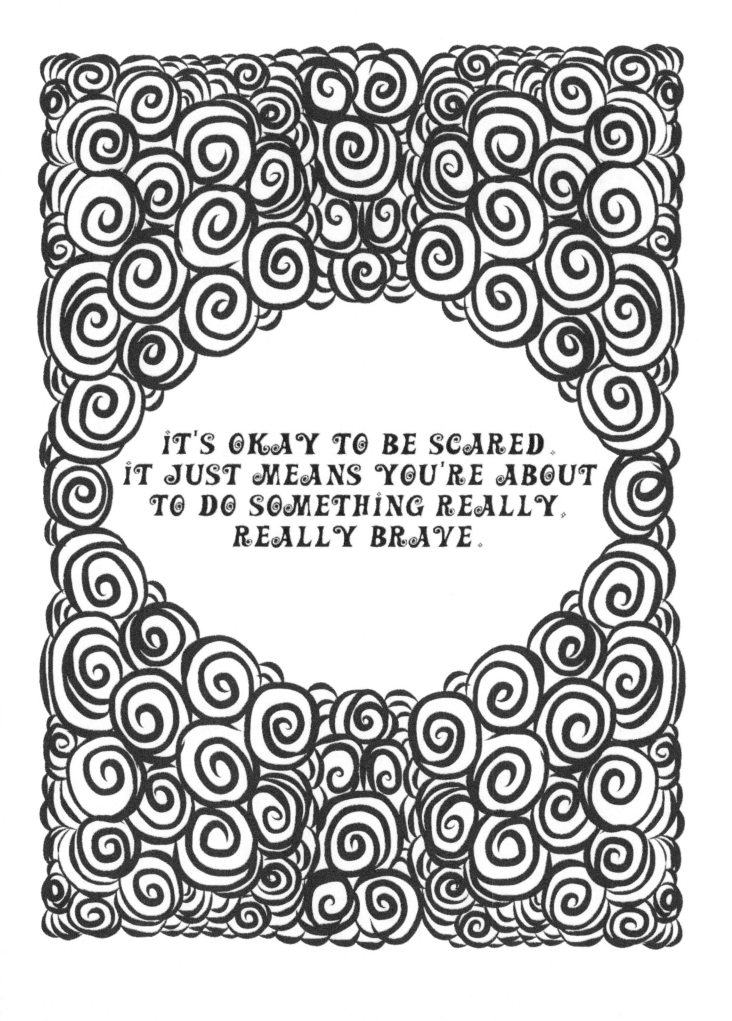

IT'S OKAY TO BE SCARED.
IT JUST MEANS YOU'RE ABOUT
TO DO SOMETHING REALLY,
REALLY BRAVE.

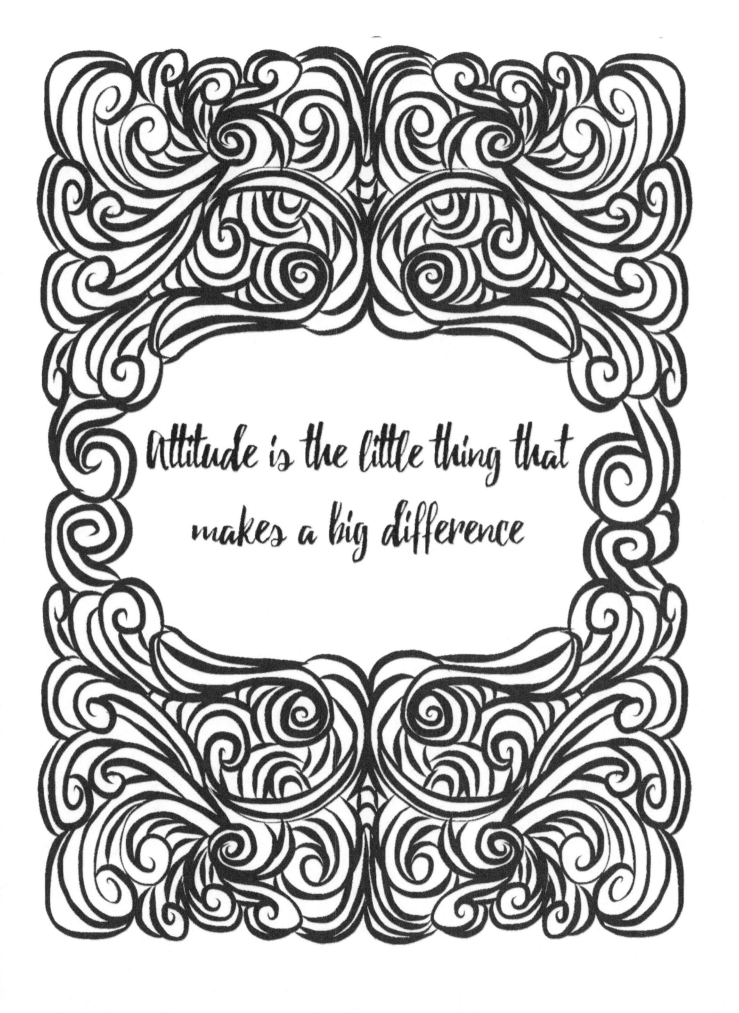

Attitude is the little thing that makes a big difference

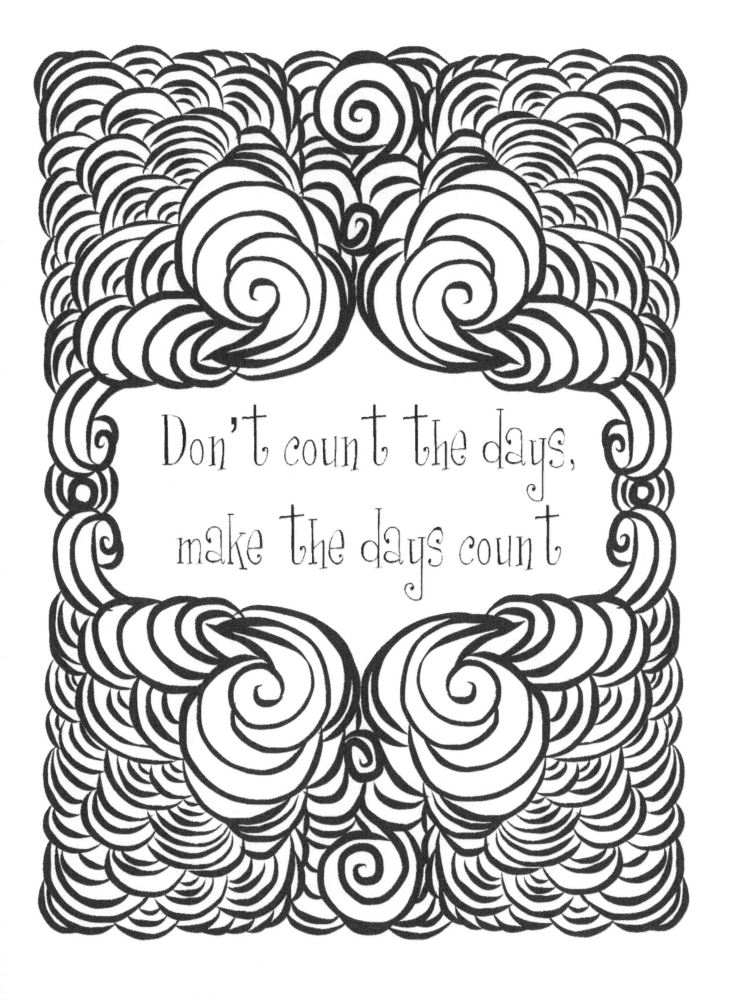

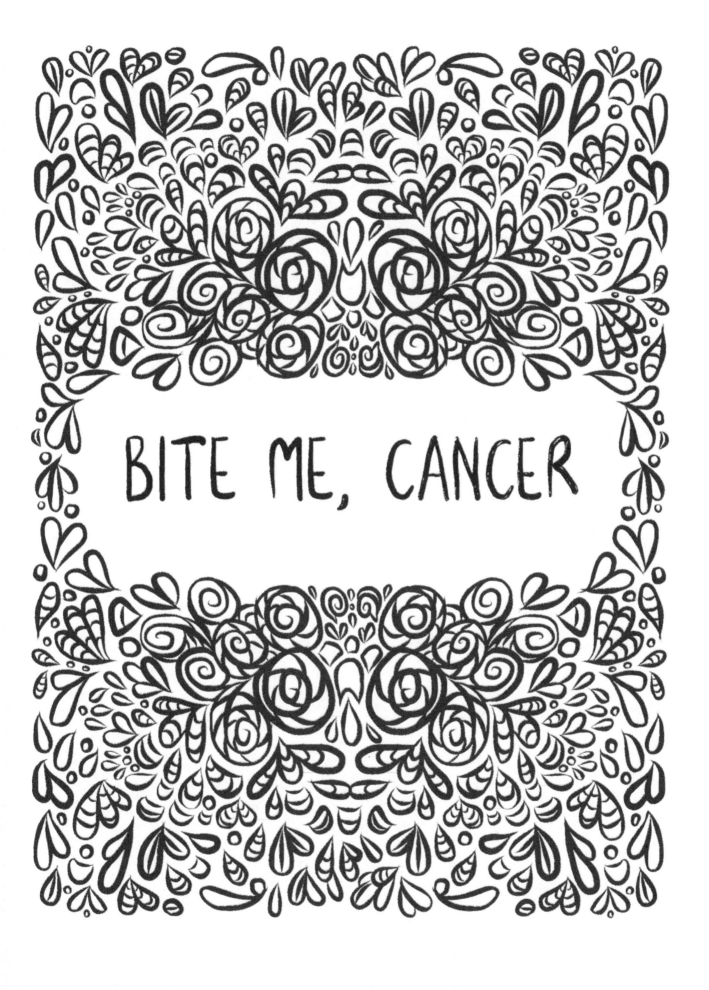

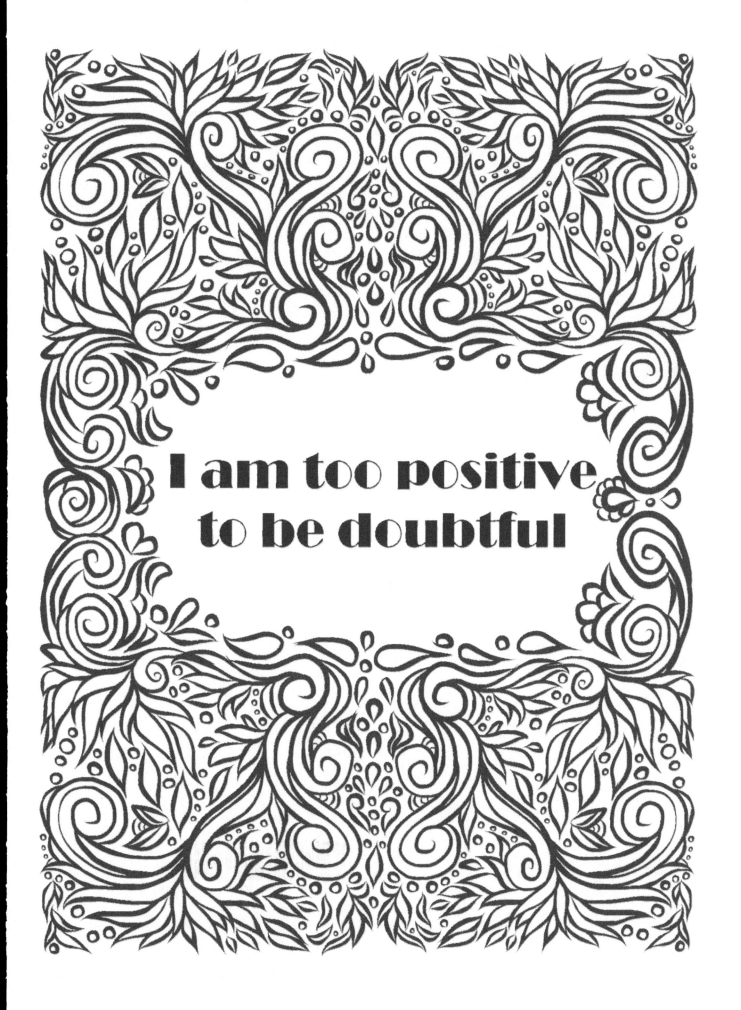

Made in the USA
Middletown, DE
03 January 2024

47172425R00038